ENHANCE YOUR CHEST CLEAVAGE AND MAKE YOUR BREASTS LOOK firmer and BIGGER with HOME EXERCISES

how to improve the appearance of your breasts:

chest cleavage adds beauty ,sex appeal and femininity to any woman!

Well shaped cleavage is a sign of robust health, good posture and beauty for both men and women.

The exercises in this book , will enhance your cleavage and you can do them anywhere at any time without any expensive equipment or the need to go to the gym!

S.ELIA

how to improve the appearance of your
breasts:

chest cleavage adds beauty ,sex appeal
and femininity to any woman!

Well shaped cleavage is a sign of robust

health, good posture and beauty for both
men and women.

Self published by S .ELIA

With Kindle Direct Publishing   @ amazon.com

Disclaimer:
This book is for information only   and is not

intended as medical advise. if you need medical advise, consult your trusted doctor for proper diagnosis and treatments.
The suggested exercises in this book are good for anybody who wants to enhance his or her cleavage by strengthening the chest muscles. However if you have any health issues with your chest or breasts, check with your health professional for proper diagnosis and treatments, before starting any exercises..

S.ELIA

CONTENTS

12) simple exercises to enhance your cleavage.

1) INTRODUCTION

I was watching a beautiful young lady on television complaining that a certain   male actor had a better cleavage than her. That woman was beautiful, attractive and sexy, but still she wanted to have a better cleavage for obvious reasons, to feel more feminine and sexy.

 So I thought, if this beautiful young lady has issues with her appearance and her cleavage, just imagine how many other women that are not as beautiful will feel about their appearances and their cleavage.

In a way she was right that some men have a bigger cleavage that some women, and that is due to the fact that exercise and work hard so that their chest muscles are well developed and they have big chest muscles that form a cleavage that many women would be envy to have.

2)What is the cleavage anyway

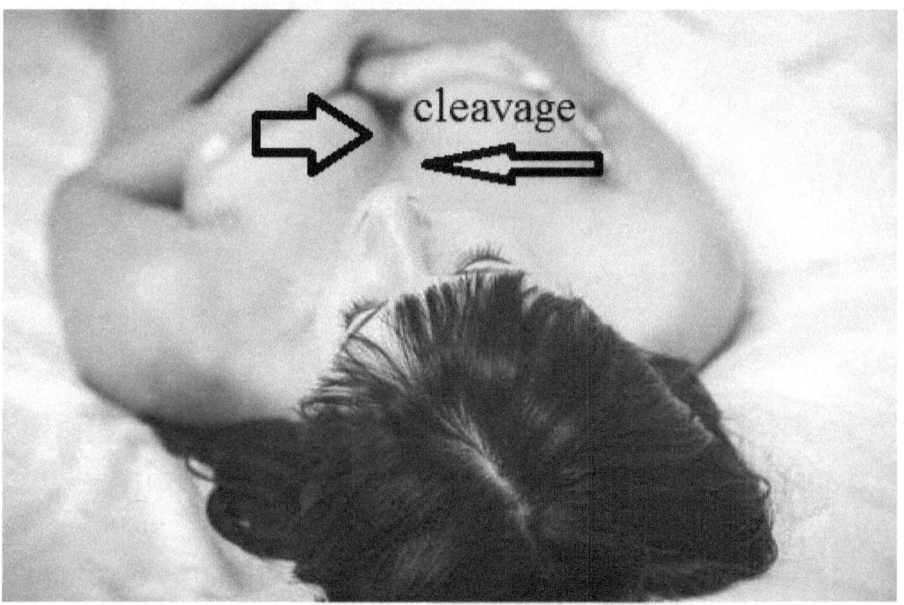

Cleavage is the area between the left and right breast over the sternum.

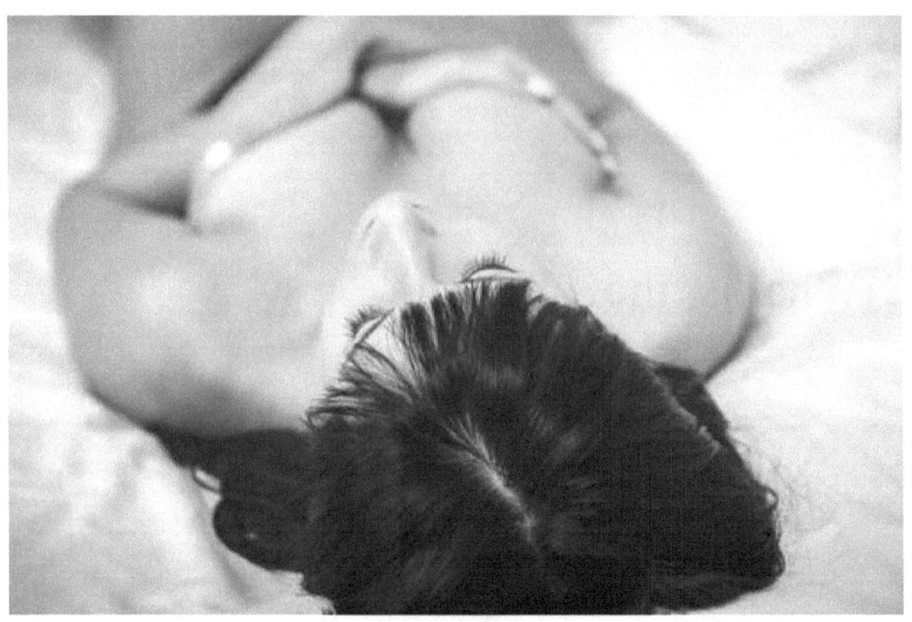

In reality, Cleavage is the exposed area between the left and right chest muscles over the sternum area and in the case of the woman the area between the breasts over the sternum, and refers only to what is visible with clothing that includes a low-cut neckline. The display of women's cleavage is considered aesthetic, sexy or erotic. Women wear clothes with low necklines garments that expose or highlight cleavage, such as ball gowns, evening gowns, lingerie, and swimwear.

 From time immemorial the women have throughout history, sought to enhance their physical attractiveness and femininity, within the context of changing fashions and cultural-specific norms of modesty of the time and place. In some religious cultures any display of cleavage may be culturally accessible, illegal or otherwise socially disapproved of.

Many women desire a bigger cleavage so that they feel more attractive, sexy and desirable.

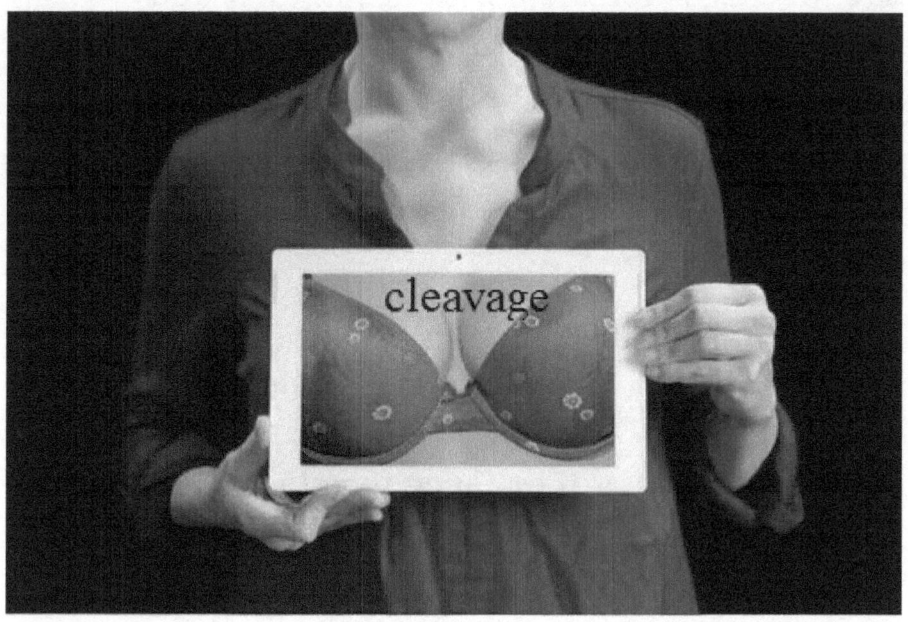

In females, a well developed cleavage depends on the condition of the chest muscles and the size of the female breast. There are millions of women who are jealous of women who have beautiful and curvaceous cleavages. Some of them even end up having surgeries to enhance their breasts and their cleavage.

It is a fact that a well developed chest cleavage, adds beauty ,sex appeal and femininity to any

**woman!**

Cleavage in men, it all depends of the condition of the big chest muscles , called , pectoral muscles, although in rare occasions there are men that actually have breasts too, called gynecomastia, due to excess female hormones in their body. **Gynecomastia is** the enlargement of the breast tissues in men due to hormonal imbalance.
**It is a fact that a well shaped cleavage is a sign of robust health, good posture and beauty for both men and women.**

In this book we are going to describe exercises that will enhance the cleavage area in both men and women.
These exercises will enhance the cleavage area , which is the area between the left and right pectoral muscles the chest over the sternum. Sternum, also know as the breastbone, is the bone in the middle of your chest where the ribs are attached forming the chest cavity.
These exercises will firm up the female breasts but it will not enlarge the breasts size , due to the fact that the female breasts are glands and not muscles.

3) chest anatomy:

In order to have a nice cleavage you have to understand the anatomy of the chest. A well formed chest will have a nice cleavage. A malformed or underdeveloped chest will not have a nice cleavage.

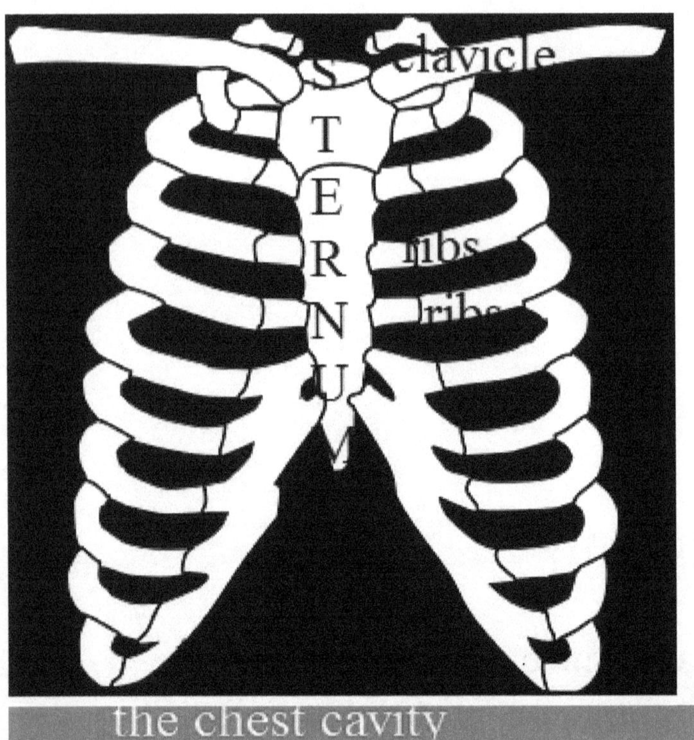

The cleavage is the area between the left and right chest pectoral muscles, over the sternum. The chest muscles are over the chest cavity , also know as the thoracic cavity, which is the second largest hollow space of the body. The thoracic cavity is enclosed by the ribs, the vertebral column, and the sternum, or breastbone, and is separated from the abdominal cavity which is the body's largest hollow space, by a muscular and membranous partition, the diaphragm.

The chest cavity contains the lungs, the middle and lower airways and the heart. The ribs are attached to the spinal column in the back and the sternum in the front.   The anterior ribcage is covered with the pectoral muscles which form the cleavage space over the sternum. In order to have a well formed cleavage

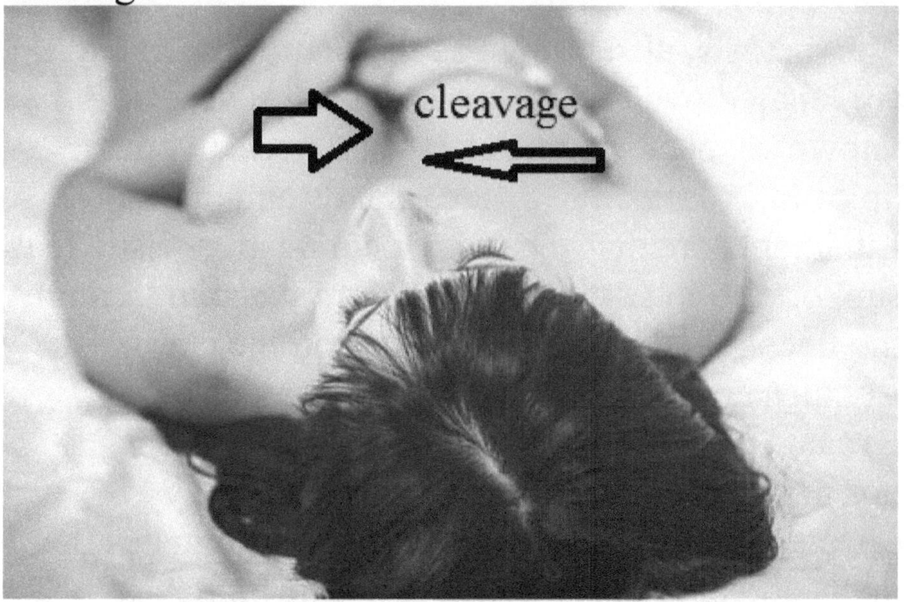

you have to have a well developed rib cage and strong healthy chest muscles. Over the chest muscles are the left and right breasts .

The breasts in men are not functional but just the breast nipples are visible.
The breasts in females are functional and they produce milk for the babies. The female breasts

come in different shapes and sizes.
The size of the female breasts and the condition of the chest muscles determines the shape and size of the cleavage.

4) breast anatomy.

The breasts, also known as the mammary glands are located over the front chest muscles also known as pectoral muscles. The **breast** is made up of fat, connective tissue, glands and ducts. Ligaments are dense bands of connective tissue that support the **breast**. They run from the skin through the **breast** and attach to muscles on the chest. Lobules are the groups of glands that make milk. **Breast** development and function depend on hormones produced by the ovaries, namely estrogen and progesterone. Estrogen elongates the ducts and causes them to create side branches. Progesterone increases the number and size of the lobules in order to prepare the breast for milk production to nourishing a baby.

Both males and females have breasts but the male breasts are not functional and produce no milk. The structure of the male breast is nearly identical to that of the female breast, except that the male breast tissue lacks the specialized lobules to produce milk.

In females the breasts **have** also a

psychological function in that it is associated with sexuality. Underdeveloped breasts or partial or complete removal, which may be necessary to treat certain diseases like breast cancer may cause significant emotional distress.

The function of the breast is to provide milk to feed the infants. Milk is produced and stored by the mammary glands and released through the mammary ducts and nipple. Infants thrive on the nutritious mother's milk.

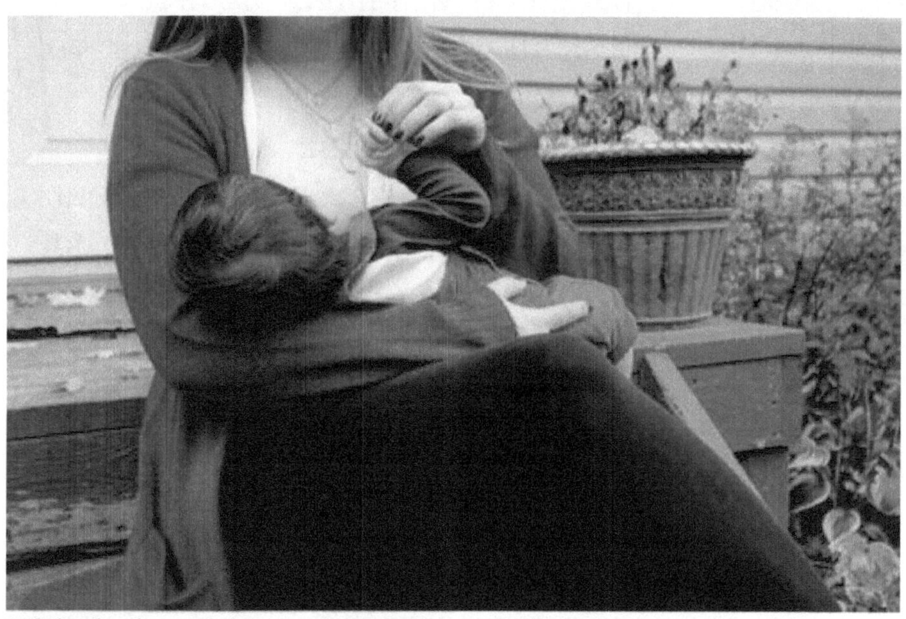

This baby enjoys the most nutritious meal of the day, his mother's breast milk, which has everything the baby needs to grow and flourish.

You cannot put a price on that! that's priceless!

5) breasts and genes

 The female breasts are not the same shape or size in all women. If you ever had the chance to walk on a crowded beach in the summer time where many women are with or without their bathing suits you will see that some women have huge breasts and others hardly have any breasts.
The breast development depends on the human genes and it runs in families. If the mother had big breasts, her daughters will have big breasts and if the mother had small breasts , her daughters will have small breasts too.
So what ever size of breasts you have, feel comfortable with your breast size and thank your genes with whatever the nature gave you. It is not the size that matter but how you feel and your health.
Women with huge breasts might look sexy and attractive but they have their own problems too !
So enjoy whatever you have and thank nature for whatever you have. Nature knows best what is suitable for you.

6)purpose of the breasts.

Nature made the breasts for one purpose and one purpose only, to produce nutritional milk to feed the infants. As long as you are able to produce enough milk to feed your infant kids that is good enough for your kids. Infants just need nutritious milk to satisfy their hunger and grow fast.
Even if you do not produce enough milk for your infant babies, do not worry and you are not alone, even women with huge breasts sometimes do not produce enough milk to satisfy the hunger of their infants.
 Fortunately now a days there is a huge variety of baby formulas for the infants which most women use for their babies even when their breasts produce enough milk to feed their babies..

7) animal breasts:

If you ever had the opportunity to visit an animal farm or the zoo you will notice that many female animals have noticeable breasts only during their pregnancy and the lactation period. Breast development in other primate females generally only occurs with pregnancy. Unlike human females, the animal females do not give that much importance to the size of their breasts and all they want is to have enough milk to feed their babies.

8)how to improve the appearance of your breasts:

The only way to improve the appearance of your breasts is to exercise the foundation of your breasts which is the chest muscles, also known as pectoral muscles. Bigger, stronger, healthier chest muscles will improve the appearance of the breasts no matter how big or how small the breasts are.
The exercises I describe in this book will help you get stronger and bigger chest muscles and will uplift and firm your breasts making the breasts look bigger and better with an enhance cleavage. All you have to do is do the exercises daily.

Another important building block to improve your breast appearance is to have a good nutritious diet.

 Perhaps this is the most important of all the requirements for your breasts and your whole health in general. You have to provide your body with all the necessary nutrients for good health.

When your body has the necessary nutrients, all parts of the body including the breasts will function properly.

Yo-yo diets , unnecessary diets or starving diets will have a detrimental effect on the health of the body and many parts of the body including the breasts will pay the consequences.

You cannot have a malnourished starving body with   good appearances. Self impose or force starvation has a detrimental effect on the body, the breasts and every other organ of the body. Some people with anorexia , which is an eating disorder, their bodies are emaciated and they are just bones and skin. All the organs of starving people are suffering including their breasts .

   A good diet providing all the nutrients for your body's need will do wonders for your health and the appearances of your chest and breast.

A good nutritional diet is essential for good health, good looks and well developed breast too.

Your eating habits should include milk and milk products. Milk is a wholesome food that can sustain life. The babies eat nothing but just drinking milk for a few months and not only survive but they flourish too.

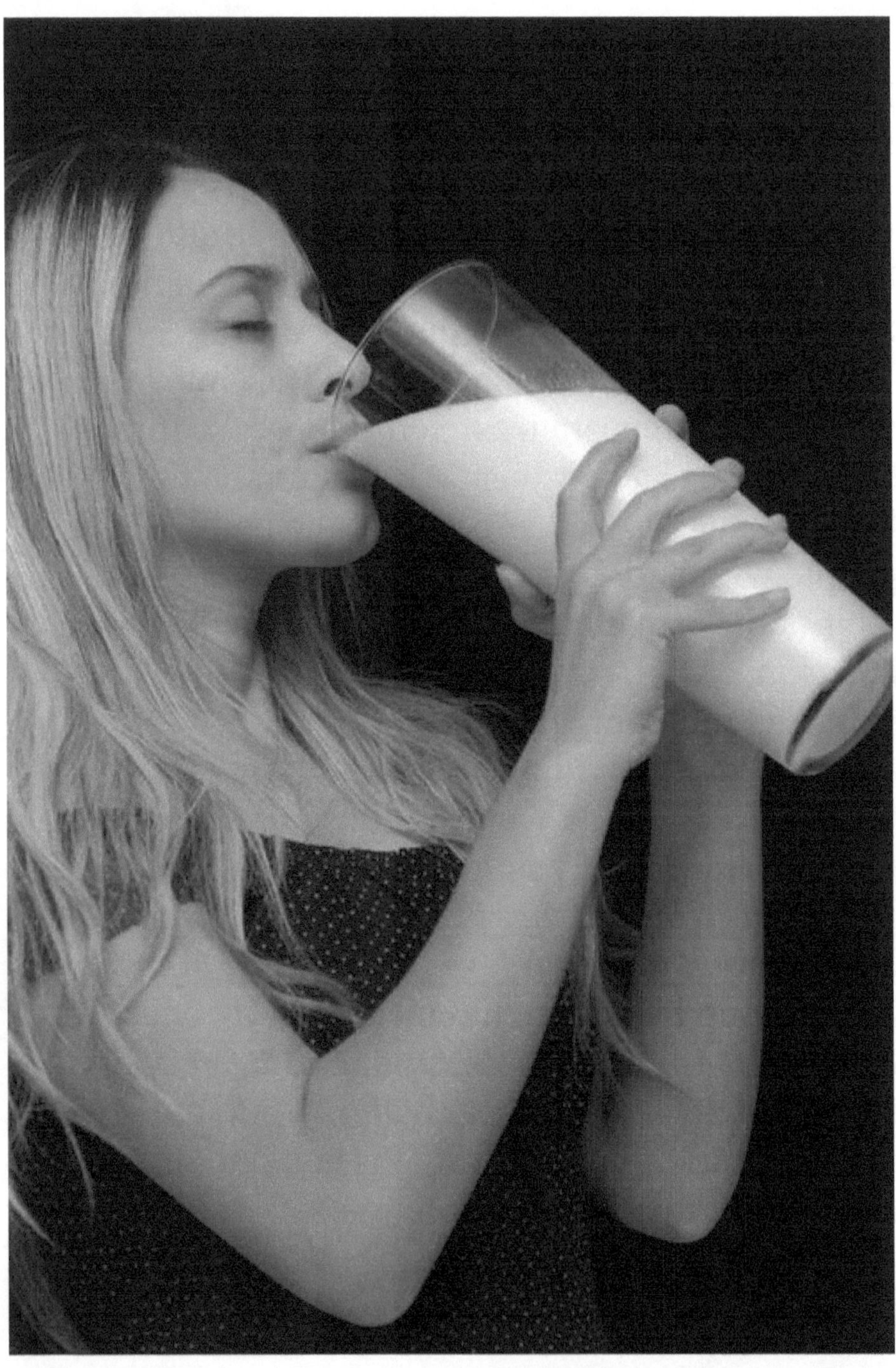

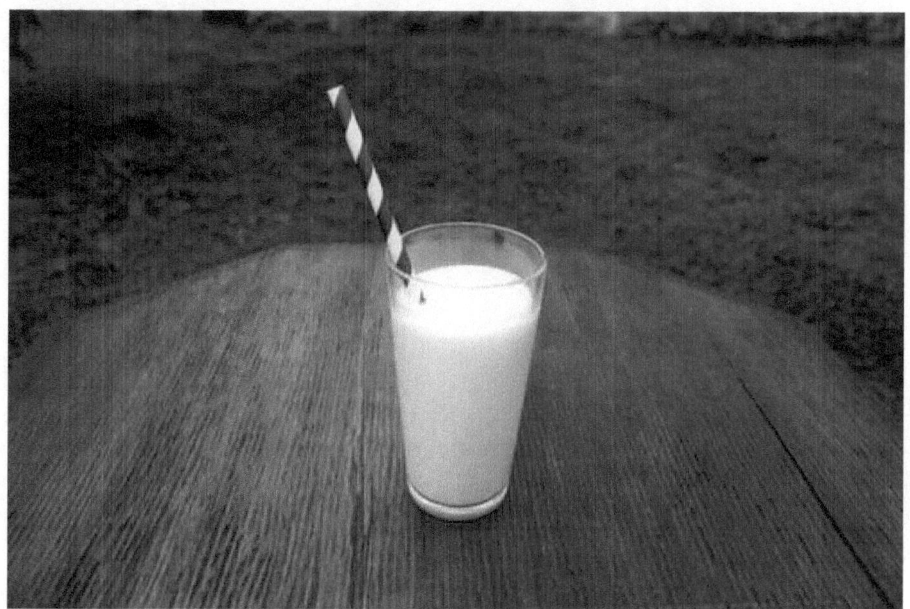

Milk is a wholesome nutritional food that can sustain life.

Another wholesome food are the eggs which have all the ingredients to develop a new life, the chick.

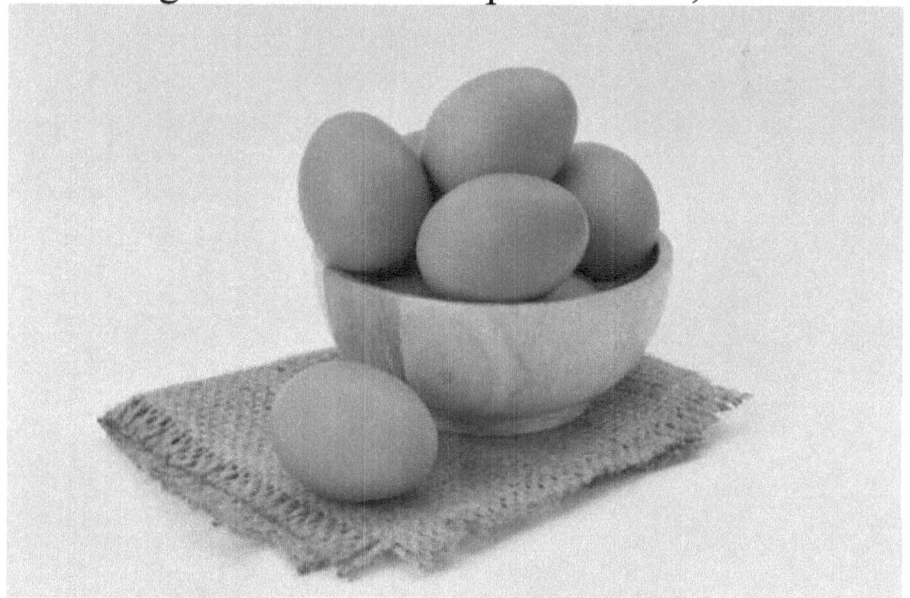

Eggs are very nutritious food.

Meat and nuts are very good sources for good nutrition.

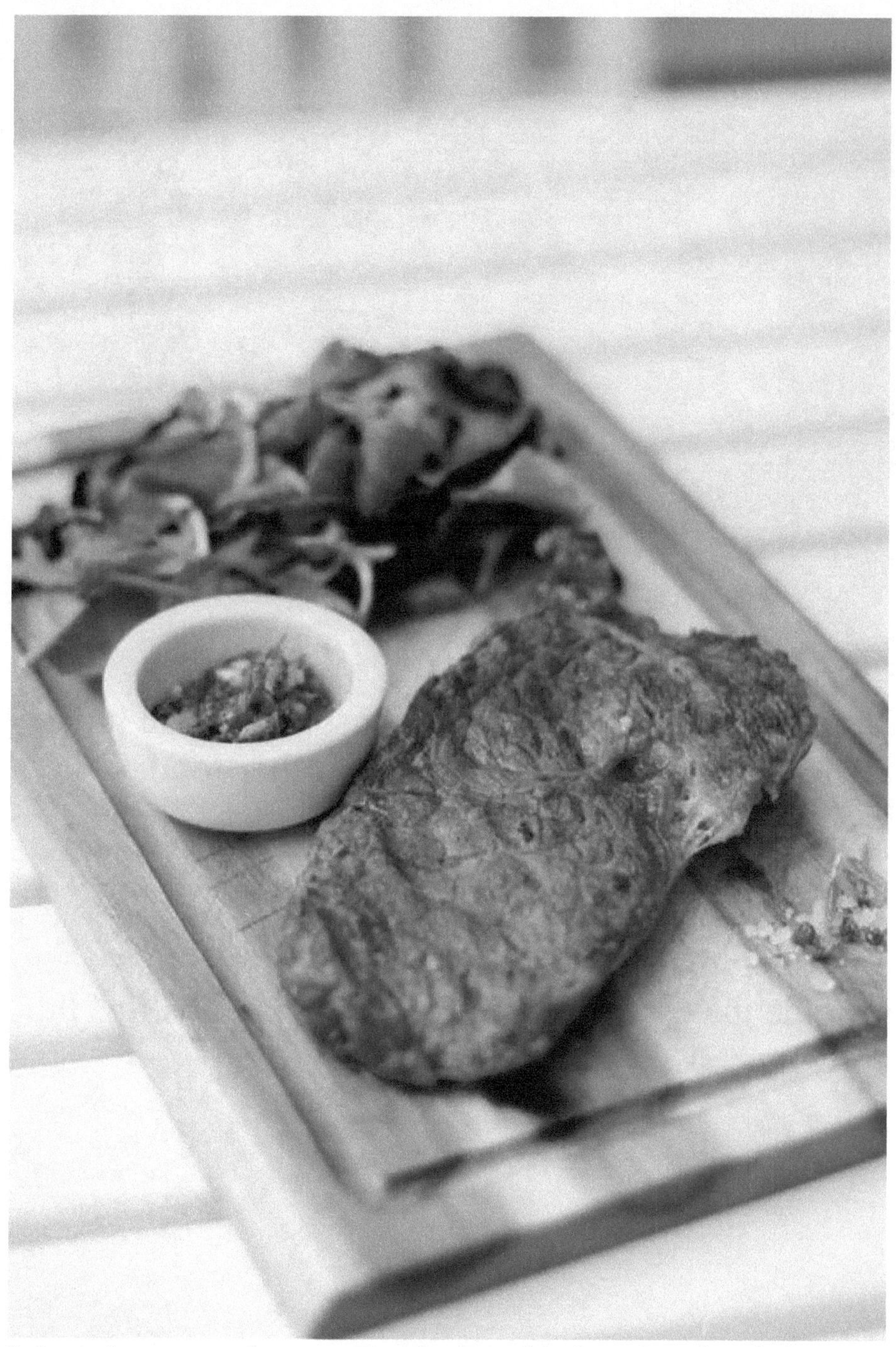

Meat is a good source of protein for the body's

protein needs.

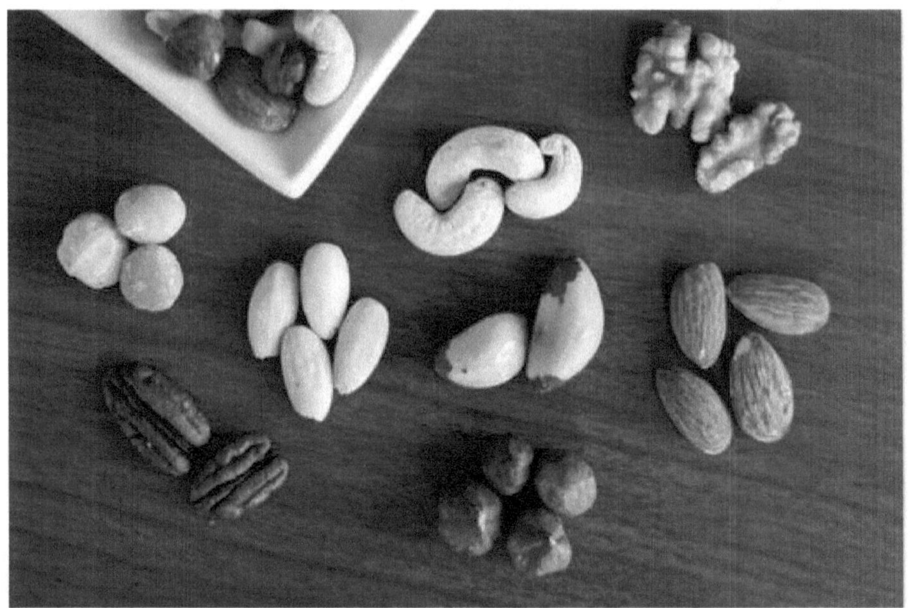

Nuts are delicious and nutritious, but if you have allergy to any of the nuts, or any other food, DO NOT EAT THEM,

You should also eat vegetables and fruits that provide the essential minerals and vitamins for the body's needs.

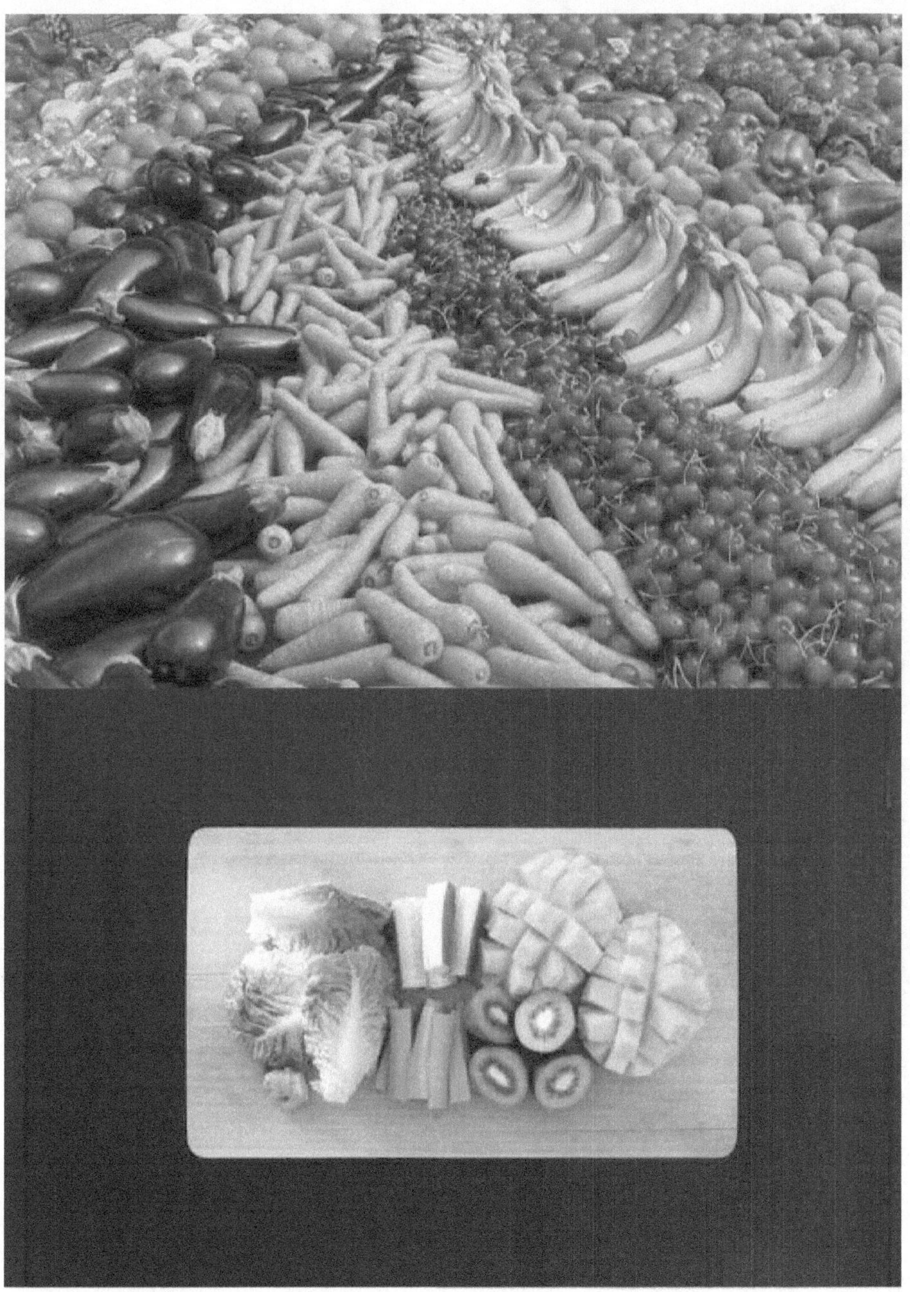

Fruits and vegetables is a good source of vitamins and minerals for the body's needs.

9)breasts in men and women

Both men and women have breasts but only the women have functional breast that really make nutritious milk for the babies.
The breasts are influenced by the hormones of the body. At puberty, the female hormones estrogens, in conjunction with growth hormone, cause breast development in female humans and to a much lesser extent in other animals. In females, it serves as the mammary gland, which produces and secretes milk to feed infants.
In males the male testosterone hormone causes the development of testes and the production of spermatozoa and inhibits the development of breasts.
If any males take estrogen hormones it will cause the breasts to enlarge something which not many males want.
If any women take testosterone they will develop facial   hair growth, something that not many women want.
Breast development in other primate females generally only occurs with pregnancy for the

production of milk for their young animal babies.

10)cleavage in men and women

Cleavage is present in both men and women but is more noticeable in women depending on the size of their breasts.

The cleavage presence in men is due to their chest muscles development from hard work or exercises. Many body builders have huge chest muscles and a very noticeable cleavage which is the envy of many women., hence the comment of that woman I saw on television, complaining that a certain actor had more cleavage than her. Cleavage in men is inconsequential and not many men pay any attention to it, or try to enhance it. It just comes naturally with hard work and strenuous exercises. In women the cleavage is formed by the chest muscles and the size of their breasts. The bigger the breasts the bigger the cleavage, especially when they wear tight low neckline dresses.

 Cleavage in women is very important and makes them feel attractive , sexy, desirable and above all self confident that they are wanted.

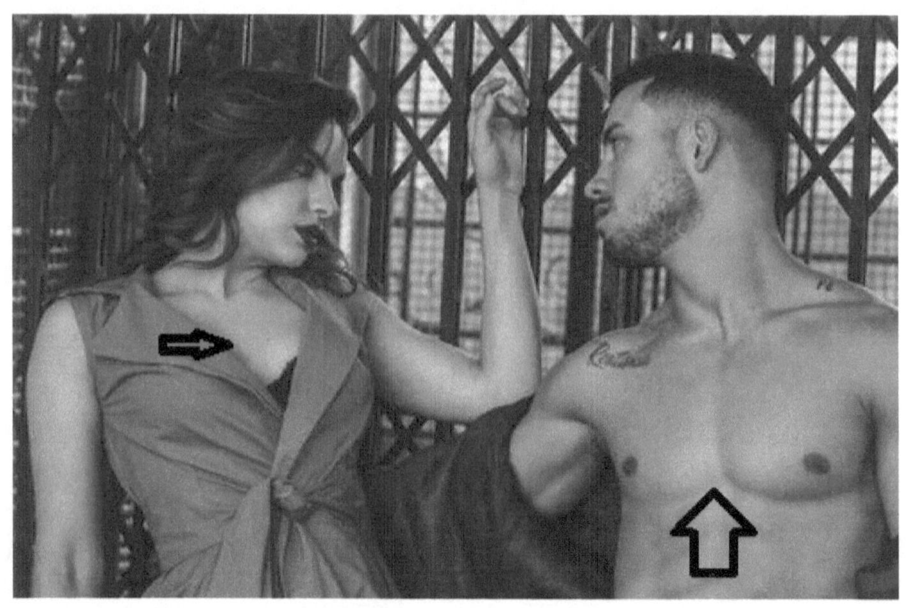

FEMALE AND MALE CLEAVAGE

Pictures of a woman and a man cleavage provided by pexels

11)how women feel about their chest's cleavage?

To many women, cleavage is very important and they try to enhance it any way they can. Some of them wear low neckline tight dresses to show off their sexy cleavage. Cleavage make them feel attractive, sexy, and boosts their self confidence as desirable.

Here is an excerpt of a woman's description how she felt about her cleavage." So, now that I actually have some amount of **cleavage** and a much better self-esteem, it makes me **feel** extremely sexy to be able to show off my chest a bit. The idea that guys are looking at me and find me attractive is a huge confidence-builder for me."

And she is right. Who can blame her, that her cleavage make her feel so good about herself? Anything that makes people feel good about themselves is a good thing.

12) simple exercises to enhance your cleavage.

There are many exercises that can enhance your cleavage, but they are time consuming and you have to use equipments or go to the gym.

The exercises I describe in this book , are more effective and you can do them anywhere at any time without any equipment or expensive gym memberships!

If you really want to enhance your cleavage you have to exercise and make your chest muscles bigger and stronger. There is no other way, you have to do the exercises, and you will reap the benefits.

Unfortunately there is no magic pill to take it and enhance your cleavage. Just the old fashion way, exercising daily two to three times a day.
Besides your cleavage benefits, you will have other health benefits too. You will have strong chest muscles, a well formed chest and a good posture. Below I will describe a few chest exercises for women that will help you to uplift your breasts and improve your cleavage. You do not need to go to a gym or any expensive equipment. You can do these exercises at home or anywhere else at any time you want.

So lets get to the exercises that will enhance your cleavage, firm up your breasts, give you a nice chest and a good posture. you will look and feel wonderful !

Disclaimer:
The exercises in this book , are exercises to improve the looks of your breasts, to be firm, look bigger and enhance your cleavage.
The breasts are glands and have no muscles to exercise to make them bigger.
The breasts are on top of the chest muscles , also know as pectoral muscles, and when you exercise

the chest muscle to make them stronger and bigger
it will have a positive effect on the breasts too.
Strong and bigger chest muscles will uplift your
breasts, making the breasts look firm and bigger
and you will have a bigger sexier cleavage, making
you look more attractive, desirable and sexy.
Bigger, stronger, healthier chest muscles will
improve the appearance of the breasts no matter
how big or how small the breasts are.
The Author

1) EXERCISE ONE: you can to this exercise
while sitting, standing or even lying down.

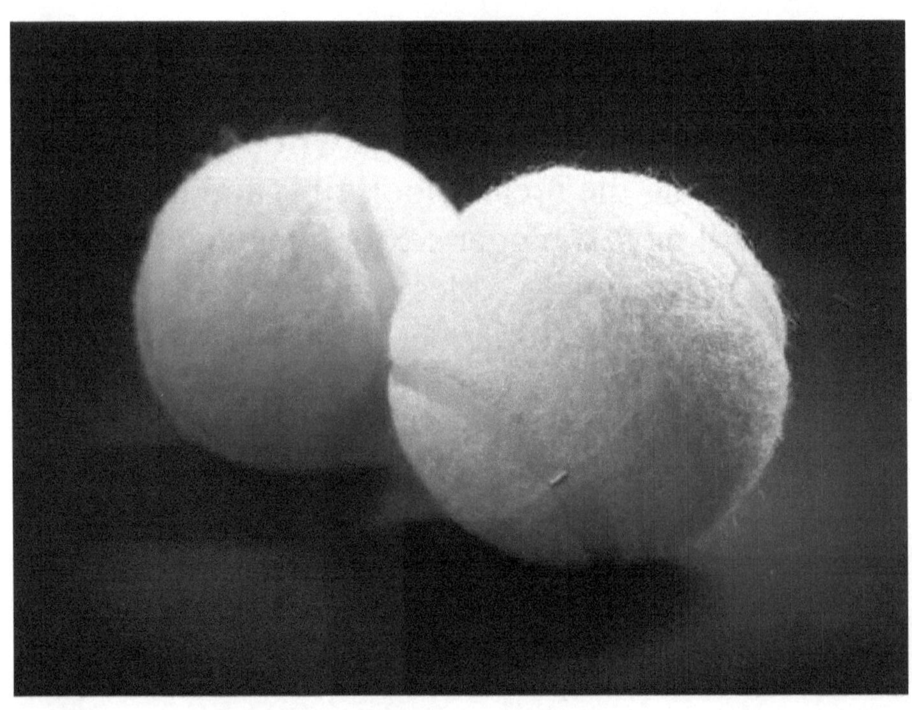

 take a tennis ball and place it between your two palms and interlock your fingers .
Bring your hands close to your chest near your cleavage area.

Squeeze the tennis ball as hard as you can to the count of three.

Relax and repeat the squeeze 5 to ten times

N.B. go easy on the exercises and do not over do it or strain yourself. With time you will be able to do more and with ease.

**While you are doing the exercises you should feel your chest muscles, also known as pectoral muscles to contract and relax.**

By repeating these exercises daily as often as possible 3 to 5 times daily and as you are getting stronger increase the repetitions, your chest muscles will get stronger and will create a nice cleavage and your breasts, no matter what their size is will get firmer and look better.
If you do not have a tennis ball, you can still do the exercises without the ball,
**just interlock your fingers, bring your hands closed to your chest over the cleavage area and press your palms against each other to the count of three, relax and repeat the exercise 5-10 times, several times during the day.**

With the tennis ball the exercises are more effective.

You can do these exercises at any time, anywhere you are, even at your work, watching television or even waiting for the bus.

N.B. this exercise is the most effective for enhancing the chest cleavage area by

<u>strengthening the chest muscles and firm and uplift your breasts.</u>

<u>2)*EXERCISE TWO:*</u> you can do this exercise while sitting standing or lying down anywhere you are at any time .

<u>Extend your arms in front of you and place your one hand over the other</u>
<u>And raise your arms above your head</u>

<u>And then lower them down in front of you</u>

<u>Repeat this exercise, raising your extended arms from the horizontal to above your head ten to twenty times</u>

And as you get stronger increase the repetitions to fifty.

<u>N.B. make sure that your bra are comfortable and do not cause any discomfort while you do this exercise.</u>

You can do this exercise at the same time when you

do the tennis ball squeeze.
This exercise uplifts and strengthens your chest muscles and will firm and uplift your breasts.

3)EXERCISE THREE: you can do this only while standing.

Stand straight with your feet about 12 inches apart.

Place your hands behind your back at the level of your sacrum (the bone that holds the pelvis together) and hold your one wrist with your other hand

While in that position bring your shoulders as back as you can without straining and hold it for the count of three and relax.

Repeat this exercises for 5-10 times.
This exercise expands, stretches and strengthens the chest muscles and by doing this exercise you will also be rewarded with a good posture!

4) exercise four

This exercise is a gentle massage of your breasts after you had a bath or a shower.

Put a few drops of virgin olive oil in you palm and rub your palms together until both palms are covered with olive oil.

With your oily right palm gently massage your left breast in a circular manner for a few seconds. Do not overdo it.

Then with your oily left palm gently massage your left breast for a few seconds.

Or you can just do gentle massage with both palms at the same time in a light circular manner. Your right palm for your right breast and your left palm for your left breast.

N.B.   when I say gentle massage , you just rub your palms gently over your breasts skin, without squeezing and definitely no deep massage of the breasts .
While you gently rubbing your breasts with your oily palms , whisper to your breasts.
" I am proud of you my tits,
make milk for my kids".

Positive affirmations, produce positive results and you should be proud of your "tits" (breasts) , no matter of their size.

Do not wipe off the oil from your breasts. Your skin will absorb the oil and will make it look good and shiny.

By doing the above exercises daily you will have the chance to strengthen your chest muscles, enhance your cleavage , uplift your breasts, and have a good posture too. You will look attractive, self confident, sexy and desirable. Good luck to all.

N.B. THE NUMBER ONE EXERCISE IS THE BEST AND THE MOST IMPORTANT, MAKE SURE YOU DO THIS ONE FOR GOOD RESULTS!

Conclusion.

It is a fact that a well developed cleavage   makes
a woman self confident, looks more attractive,
desirable and sexy. It also gives her the feeling that
she is feminine, attractive , desirable and wanted.
Many women due to heredity and their genes have
well developed breasts and cleavage. that's in
their genes. Other s do not have big breasts and
cleavage   and that is the way it is, that's in their
genes too.
With the   exercises I describe in this book, many
women can develop strong, healthy chest muscles
that will enhance their cleavage uplift their
breasts , since the breasts are over the chest
muscles, and they will have a good posture too.
All these qualities , will give them self
confidence, feeling attractive, sexy and desirable.
And that is exactly what every woman wants.
All they have to do, is to do the exercise daily at
their own convenience, at any place , at any time..

References;
All pictures are from the pexels and Pixabay websites which provide free pictures without any attribution and I thank them for that.
Here is their description.
"Thousands of royalty **free images**. Search through thousands of royalty **free images** on **Pexels**. You can use all **images** on **Pexels** for **free**, even for commercial use. All **images** are completely royalty **free**. How is that possible? All **images** on **Pexels** are licensed under the Creative Commons Zero license. Feel **free** to use them for any project you want "...

From the inside cover:
After reading this book and you no longer need it,
give it to someone else to read it and benefit from
the knowledge in this book.
Knowledge is to be shared for the benefit of all.

The only reason why Books are written is to convey information for the benefit of all.
You can also write a good review of this book, encouraging other people to read it and benefit from the knowledge in this book

From the author:

The exercises I describe in this book , are effective and you can do them anywhere at any time without any expensive equipment or the need to go to the gym!

A well developed chest cleavage adds beauty ,sex appeal and femininity to any woman!
A well shaped cleavage is a sign of robust health, good posture and beauty for both men and women. With the   exercises I describe in this book, many women can develop strong, healthy chest muscles that will enhance their cleavage, uplift their breasts , since the breasts are over the chest muscles, and they will have a good posture too. All these qualities , will give them self confidence, feeling attractive, sexy and desirable. It is my sincere hope that all the women that do these exercises, will be rewarded handsomely with a beautiful chest, and a well developed cleavage .

For the back cover:

Are you sick and tired of looking at your worn out
cleavage?
Read this book to learn how exercises can
enhance your cleavage.
This book will show you which exercises are the
best to enhance your cleavage and uplift your
breasts.
Are you willing to exercise to improve your
cleavage, your health and your self esteem?
Do you want to feel attractive, sexy, self confident
and desirable with a well developed cleavage? all
you have to do is to buy this book and start
exercising to enhance your cleavage, uplift your
breasts and your emotions..